ALL

IRRITABLE
BOWEL
SYNDROME

ALL ABOUT

IRRITABLE BOWEL SYNDROME

David Potterton
ND, MRN, MNIMH

CONSULTANT MEDICAL HERBALIST
AND REGISTERED NATUROPATH

foulsham

LONDON · NEW YORK · TORONTO · SYDNEY

foulsham

Bennetts Close, Cippenham, Berks, SL1 5AP

ISBN 0-572-02165-8

Printed in Great Britain by St Edmundsbury Press Ltd,
Bury St Edmunds, Suffolk.
Phototypeset by Typesetting Solutions, Slough, Berks.

Preface

Herbal medicine has been used since time immemorial for the relief of illness — not least for gastrointestinal problems. Today, after nearly 50 years of a national health service which dispenses drugs for almost every ill, herbal medicine is as popular as ever.

Many people who fall ill, initially treat themselves rather than go to their doctor, and this is reflected in the huge pharmaceutical business devoted to "otc" or over-the-counter medicines, the expenditure on which now amounts to about £950 million a year.

It was recently reported that over a two-week period most people suffer five different symptoms. Forty per cent of these go completely untreated, about ten per cent are treated with home remedies, twenty-four per cent with an over-the-counter medicine, thirteen per cent with a prescription medicine *already* obtained from the family doctor, while thirteen per cent of symptoms are worrying enough for people to seek medical advice.

Of those who turn to what is now called "complementary medicine" a significant number use herbal medicines from health stores and other retail outlets.

A large number of people regularly consult qualified practitioners of herbal medicine and receive an on-the-spot herbal prescription made up in the practitioner's own dispensary. The advantages of this is that they can expect to receive a medicine specially made up for them as an individual, after a proper consideration of their symptoms and following any necessary examination or investigation.

Interestingly, many other "alternative" medicine practitioners often recommend herbal medicines to their patients, despite the fact that they have received little or no formal training in this branch of medicine.

This is borne out by the large number of people who telephone herbalists requesting a particular herb recommended by "their therapist".

My view, and that of my colleagues in the National Institute of Medical Herbalists, is that self-treatment with herbs for an undiagnosed condition is inadvisable, but that where the condition is a simple one and has been properly diagnosed, a measure of self treatment is acceptable provided the medicines used are obtained from a reliable supplier.

Indeed, it has been the practice of families to treat illnesses themselves all down the centuries. But herbalists consider it to be unethical for those not qualified in herbal medicine — whether they be practitioners or not — to treat others, as this will result in second-rate treatment.

However, of all the ills that afflict mankind, it is probably those that affect the gastrointestinal tract, such as flatulence, indigestion, constipation, biliousness, and irritable bowel, that are mostly self-treated and, indeed, most successfully treated with herbal medicines.

The aim of this book is to inform and explain irritable bowel syndrome to those who have been diagnosed as suffering from this condition and to suggest how it, and closely allied disorders, may be helped by herbal and naturopathic treatment.

It is strongly emphasised, however, that should any doubts about treatment arise it is advisable to seek professional help from a qualified herbal or naturopathic practitioner. This book is not a replacement for proper medical care and should not be regarded as such.

Contents

Introduction

Irritable bowel syndrome (IBS) is one of the commonest diagnoses given to patients attending gastroenterology clinics. The diagnosis usually follows the failure of a consultant surgeon to find "anything wrong" in a patient complaining of bowel symptoms, most commonly alternating constipation and diarrhoea, often with pain in the lower bowel.

This may reflect the fact that we as a nation are said to be over-sensitive about the function of our bowels and quickly report to physicians any change in bowel habit.

It may also reflect uncertainty about the disease among family doctors as they appear to be ready to refer patients to consultants for internal investigations, such as barium meal, enema and proctoscopy, when a few doses of bran appear either not to cure the condition, or to exacerbate it.

Estimates of the prevalence of irritable bowel syndrome in the community at large vary considerably, but it is thought that at least one person in 14 in Britain suffers from it. This includes those who do not "worry the doctor" about it.

It occurs more often in women than in men — again estimates vary but the most reliable seem to indicate a ratio of about 2:1. It can also occur in children and in this age group it seems to affect the sexes about equally.

The over-70s may also suffer with IBS, but the concern here is that elderly people whose bowel function suddenly changes may have a more serious underlying condition, if only because the prevalence of serious disease increases with age. Therefore, extra vigilance is required with the elderly to exclude the possibility of, for example, inflammatory bowel disease or a tumour.

It is advisable for anyone over the age of 55 with IBS to be followed up by their practitioner at regular intervals, even when a serious disease is initially excluded. This is because bowel cancer is a highly preventable disease if a good wholesome diet is taken and proper screening tests are carried out.

In Germany and the United States it is not uncommon for business executives to have as a "fringe benefit" an annual health screen which includes faecal tests and endoscopy in order to rule out early cancer. This is seen as being as important, if not more so than providing them with a company car.

The UK lags behind in this respect, not only through lack of health education, but also because there has been an over-reliance on a "free" national health service, which cannot hope to provide everything that every individual needs.

Unfortunately, a health screen that costs relatively little for an individual or a company if undertaken privately, would be horrendously expensive if the NHS had to foot the bill for everyone — and so it is not done on a routine basis.

Medical herbalists and naturopaths, however, are trained to give dietary advice and to perform faecal and other tests, although they do, as do general practitioners, rely on hospital services, for the results of more sophisticated investigations. However, when we realise that irritable bowel is in the main a dietary disease, that most cases are preventable, but that most patients (up to 70 per cent) seen by most gastroenterologists have symptoms of it, it is obvious that a great deal of the nation's money and resources are being wasted on this condition.

By contrast, following a proper diet and treatment with herbal medicines is relatively cheap and will lead to an improved level of health and wellbeing. Used correctly, herbs generally have no side-effects, are not addictive and do not require ever-increasing dosages to maintain their effect.

WORDS OF CAUTION

Herbal medicines are generally safe, but they are not without their contraindications. Therefore:

1. Never take any herbal medication during pregnancy without advice from a qualified practitioner.

2. Do not treat babies and young children, or the very elderly without obtaining professional advice as dosages are much more critical.

3. Do not take herbal medicines if you are also taking medicines from your own doctor, as the two may interact.

4. Do not self treat if you are suffering from a liver condition or heart disease.

5. Always use herbs from reputable suppliers, but preferably from a medical herbalist, rather than gathering them from the wild.

Note: Because it is recognised that there are contra-indications and that individuals may react differently to herbal remedies, the author and publishers emphasise that they cannot be held liable for any adverse effects caused by self-treatment with any of the remedies mentioned in this book. Self-treatment must be undertaken according to the individuals's own judgement.

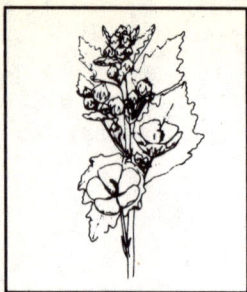

Marshmallow

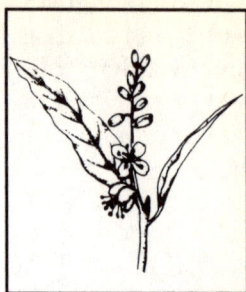

Laurel

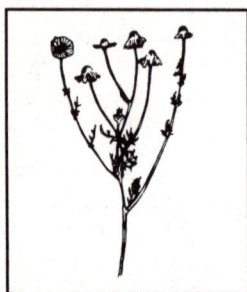

Chamomile

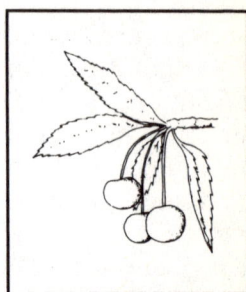

Wild Cherry

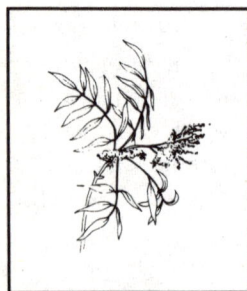

Manna

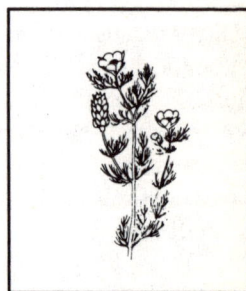

Helebore, False

Chapter 1

Irritable Colon
Identifying the Disease

It appears to be a great cause of frustration among gastroenterologists that more than half of all patients that they investigate have no organic cause to explain their symptoms, that is, they have no pathology.

Even though patients do not feel well they are often told that there is nothing wrong with them — that they are perfectly healthy. This is supposed to reassure the patient. But any frustration felt by the consultant is merely passed on to the patient who feels there is nothing that can be done to ease his complaint.

In my practice we consistently explain to patients that gastroenterological disease is more often due to malfunction, or an altered function of body systems than to specific pathology – in other words there is no gross pathological disease which can be directly observed by the doctor through an endoscope or some other instrument.

Thus, although irritable bowel syndrome is said to be the commonest disease to affect the intestinal tract of Western man, it is in many instances a last-resort label.

It is the consultant's job to rule out conditions such as bowel cancer, diverticulitis, mucous colitis, ulcerative colitis, Crohn's disease, and proctitis. Once he has done this, he tends to conclude that the patient has an irritable bowel.

"The problem is," a family doctor told me, "we don't have a simple, specific diagnostic test for irritable bowel. And we do not know the exact pathophysiology involved."

So faced with a patient complaining of abdominal pain

13

and a change in bowel habit — either alternating constipation and diarrhoea, or diarrhoea alone — doctors are apt to try out a few drugs and treatments first and will probably enquire: "Are you taking bran?" And when that fails they refer the sufferer to the nearest gastroenterology department for investigation.

The consultant may then offer antispasmodic drugs, or believing that there really is nothing wrong with the patient except undue worry about bowel function, gives tranquillisers or antidepressants ... not really a logical medical approach and one which most people would rather avoid.

THE STRESS CONNECTION

It is true to say, however, that a significant number of IBS patients do also complain of symptoms related to stress, such as fatigue, depression, anxiety, inability to sleep, and marital and emotional problems.

It is not clear whether stress alone causes irritable bowel, but there is no doubt that it can exacerbate it. Individuals seem to respond to stress rather differently. Some people immediately go off their food when they face stress, while others tend to eat more as a form of emotional compensation. Stress can inhibit digestion with resultant constipation or it can trigger attacks of diarrhoea. Where an emotional problem has been identified herbal medicine, plus one-to-one counselling, can be very helpful.

The frustration of the gastroenterologist in not being able to find anything wrong with the IBS sufferer merely confirms the views of the herbalists and naturopaths. In most cases, there is nothing dreadfully wrong with the sufferer. It is just that the body, or more specifically, the intestinal tract, is being used wrongly. The term irritable bowel explains very little. It is just the latest fashionable label for it.

Doctors have given various names to irritable bowel for centuries. It has masqueraded under a whole list of different descriptions, often depending on the main interest of the doctor involved.

The condition has been known as membraneous enteritis, which referred to the fact that some patients noted mucous in their stools. It has also, and still is, confused with mucous colitis, by many physicians. However mucous colitis and ulcerative colitis are inflammatory bowel diseases and should be regarded as separate conditions from irritable bowel. IBS has also been called muco-membraneous colitis, mucous colic, enteralgia, nervous diarrhoea, spastic colitis, spastic colon, spastic constipation and enterospasm.

HORMONES?

It is interesting what lengths orthodox researchers will go to in the pursuit of not finding out much of value.

For example, work demonstrating that the hormone cholecystokinin injected into patients with the irritable bowel syndrome made their symptoms worse caused a flurry of excitement because it was said it could explain why sufferers complain of symptoms after eating.

The hormone, you see, is released in response to the ingestion of food.

But medical herbalists and naturopaths are likely to view such findings with scepticism, because natural treatments based on commonsense and observation work successfully in most cases where the sufferer is willing to alter his artificial life-style and diet.

LACTOSE INTOLERANCE

Now I emphasise *in most cases*, because there are a few other possible causes of irritable bowel syndrome, including malabsorption of the lactose in milk. This intolerance to milk sugar can cause diarrhoea and a noisy, distended and painful abdomen, and probably accounts for about ten per cent of all cases.

It is often overlooked by family doctors and is a good example of why it is absurd to prescribe antispasmodic drugs and tranquillisers, instead of taking the time to find out what is actually responsible for the symptoms.

SYMPTOMS

Let's take a closer look at the symptoms of IBS. The urge to empty the bowel may occur with such frequency that it disrupts normal life. Visits to the toilet may start very early in the morning. But some patients may go to the toilet only once a day.

The pain, which affects most patients is usually low down, cramping or colicky, and may be relieved or made worse by the passing of stools. These are often described as being small, hard and ribbon-like. In addition there may be heartburn, flatulence and nausea. Some patients pass mucous with their stools, but unless they also have haemorrhoids, should not pass blood.

SPASTIC COLON

Another cause of irritable bowel is chronic abuse of laxatives. Simple constipation should ideally be treated by changing to a healthier diet, but many sufferers thinking that they are taking the easy way out, use laxatives that irritate the muscles of the intestine.

After years of indulging in this habit the bowel alternates between constipation and diarrhoea because it will only work when given the laxative.

Another name for this type of irritable bowel is 'spastic colon'.

It has long been said that all bowels are irritable and all bowels are irritated because if one eats the right food the colon is automatically stimulated to empty itself. Almost everyone during the course of their life will experience the symptoms of irritable bowel. It is only when the symptoms persist unduly that they are interpreted as actual disease.

WHOLE PERSON

In my practice the condition is regarded as a dysfunction of the entire person. On questioning sufferers will quite often complain of other problems such as insomnia, nervous and physical exhaustion, dizzy spells, headaches, migraine, cardiac irregularities, painful urination, vaginal discharge and anal irritation.

While orthodox physicians may write these off as psychological symptoms of no clinical significance, I would certainly consider whether they and the bowel condition were manifestations of allergy due to a deficient immune system, which in turn was the consequence of an improper diet.

People with irritated bowel will have their symptoms aggravated by stress situations related to their marital life, children, or finances. There may be emotional conflict, anxiety, loneliness, exhaustion from overwork, or a cancer phobia. And it is true that any kind of psychological stress will intensify the normal contractions of the intestine.

17

In addition to dietary advice, therefore, the sufferer may need counselling or psychotherapy, rather than tranquillisers and antidepressant drugs which merely mask the symptoms.

CORRECT DIET

What is the correct diet?

This is where a note of warning may be sounded. I do not recommend just adding bran to the diet which many physicians are apt to do, because bran may exacerbate the symptoms causing increased flatulence which balloons out the colon giving more pain.

Neither do I recommend putting the sufferer on to a fast to rest the colon or to see whether food allergy is involved.

It is essential that the bowel be kept working because it is more natural for it to work. The residue from undigested food passing through the colon provides it with its most natural environment.

At the start of treatment it is best to reduce the intake of flatulent foods such as nuts, fruit peel, pips, skins and seeds. I even recommend that tomatoes are skinned before use.

I also advise the sufferer to avoid compressed foods, like cream crackers, which can be irritating to a sensitive intestine, and any foods which are seen to pass through the colon undigested.

Because the basic cause of the condition is associated with the chronic ingestion of fibre deficient food, such as refined sugar, white bread, fancy cakes and biscuits, white pasta and confectionery, these must be excluded if a long term recovery is to be expected.

What is there left to eat?

That is usually the first question asked which really proves that the diet has been at fault.

The answer is to increase the intake of pulpy, soft fibrous foods which will soothe the inflamed and irritated gut.

Examples of these are fruits and vegetables such as boiled potato and carrots, marrows and melons, aubergines and avocados, boiled beetroot, baked banana and ripe peeled apples and pears.

Wholewheat bread and cereals should be included because they are a natural source of bran.

ALLERGY

In cases where allergy is suspected the protein foods —e.g. meat, fish, cheese, milk, eggs and butter — are best rotated with one day being kept protein free. This five-day rotation is useful in the detection of allergy, or sensitivity to food, because allergies most commonly involve one or more of these proteins. Eating, say cheese, only once in five days allows time for symptoms to recede if one is allergic to it.

In non-allergic cases I recommend a reduction in meat eating in favour of a higher intake of fish which is more easily digested. Poor digestion of the fat in meat due to insufficient bile tends to make the bowels loose.

As symptoms improve more foods are added to the diet one by one, the aim being to exclude those which obviously irritate the bowel, but to achieve as near normal a diet as possible.

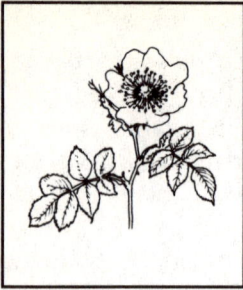

Dog Rose

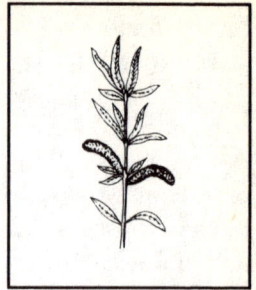

Willow, White

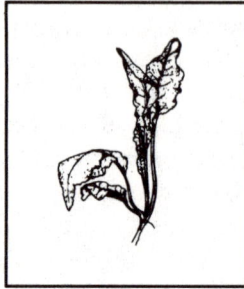

Horseradish

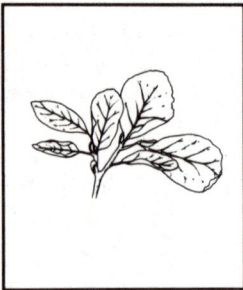

Witch Hazel

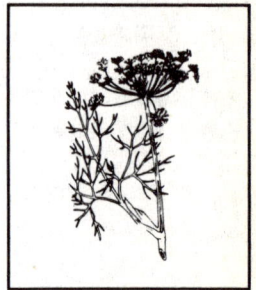

Dill

Chapter 2

The Role of Herbal Medicines

Because the person with an acute irritable colon feels that everything they eat upsets them, the use of herbal medicines is encouraged to tone up the digestive organs, to deal with concomitant conditions such as headaches or depression, to reduce inflammation and pain, to induce rest, and to assist in the absorption of nutrients from the digestive tract.

While home treatment may be successful, many cases need the support and skill of an understanding practitioner because of the individual nature of treatment from the point of view of counselling, allergies, bowel symptoms and choice of herbal medicines.

A herbal prescription will vary from person to person, but among the basic remedies that might be used for short-term treatment is oil of peppermint (Mentha piperita), which is a potent antispasmodic of the smooth muscle found in the bowel, and has local analgesic effects.

Peppermint herb has been used for centuries to allay nausea, flatulence and vomiting, and as an infants' cordial.

Pliny records that the Greeks and Romans crowned themselves with peppermint at their feasts and that it was used along with other mints by the ancient Greek physicians. It found its way into the London Pharmacopoeia in 1721.

The essential oil is probably one of the most important to be used therapeutically. It is also widely used in the production of confectionery and toothpastes. Menthol, the chief constituent, is responsible for most of the therapeutic action.

A clinical trial with peppermint oil in an enteric-coated capsule showed it to be superior to placebo in relieving irritable bowel symptoms.

Taken in capsule form the oil is not released until it has passed the stomach and, therefore, its effect on the bowel is enhanced.

In the trial at the University of Wales, patients who had previously undergone other treatments for the condition without success were given peppermint oil capsules designed to dissolve in the mid-to-terminal ileum.

The most common response from the patients was that the capsules reduced abdominal pain, although some symptoms, such as diarrhoea, were not affected.

CARMINATIVES

Carminatives such as aniseed, fennel, and liquorice help to reduce flatulence and are soothing to the lining of the stomach and intestinal tract.

Marshmallow root is emollient and stimulates healing.

Remedies that stimulate bile production like dandelion root may also be incorporated into the medicine when required.

Powdered ginger is a useful standby for nausea, flatulence and spasms of the colon and should be administered in doses of between 10 and 20 grains. Ginger is added to purgative medicines to prevent griping pains and, therefore, its use in painful conditions of the bowel is adequately borne out.

Cinnamon can also be given in small doses to reduce nausea and flatulence.

INFUSIONS

For domestic purposes it is recommended that herbs be taken by infusion — about one teaspoonful of the dried herb to one cup of boiling water. Other excellent remedies that can be taken this way are meadowsweet, rosemary and chamomile. Honey can be added to the infusion to increase palatability.

The approach outlined, particularly if it is managed by a competent herbalist, should yield satisfying results within a few weeks.

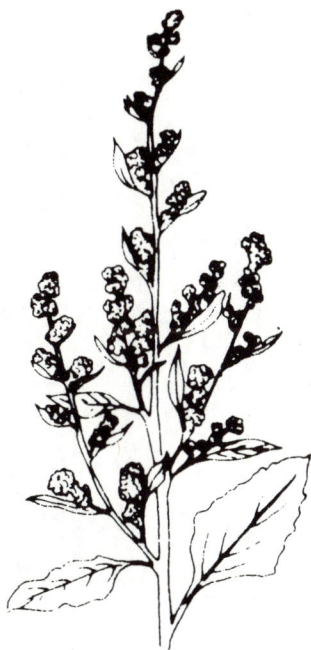

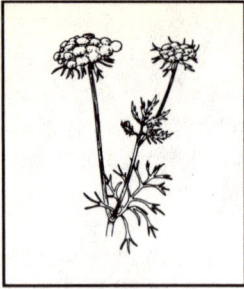

Wild Carrot

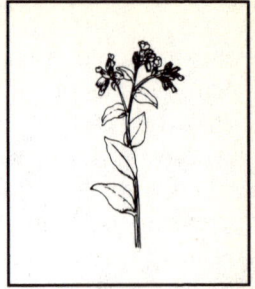

Lungwort

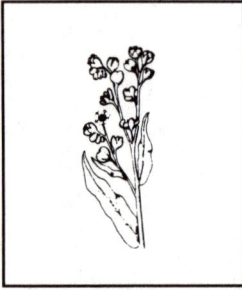

Houndstongue

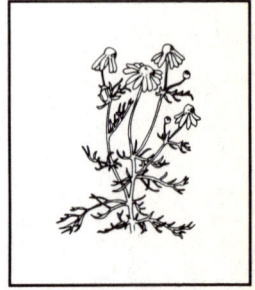

Chamomile
(German)

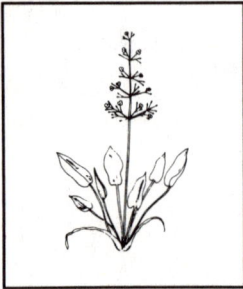

Water Plantain

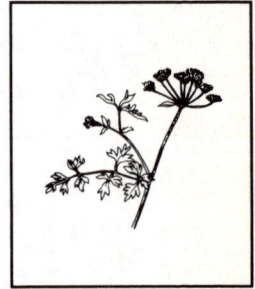

Water Dropwort
(Poisonous)

Chapter 3

Constipation
Why it resists treatment

Naturopaths and herbalists have written extensively for years on the role that diet plays in chronic constipation; and the importance of dietary fibre has been emphasised in many health education programmes during the past decade with ever-increasing success.

People with irritable bowel syndrome, however, may not find their constipation resolved simply by switching from their much-loved rice crispies to a bowel of bran flakes and there may be several reasons for this.

A more normal bowel motion and a daily habit will be achieved only if an increase in fibre is accompanied by an increase in fluid intake. Failure to take note of this may simply result in a patient's stools becoming harder and more difficult to pass.

If the sufferer has a wheat intolerance then increasing wheat fibre in the diet will only exacerbate the problem.

Patients who do not improve after making the usual changes from white to wholemeal bread and so on should be encouraged to increase other sources of fibre in their diet such as fruit, vegetables, brown rice and pulses.

If there is a disturbance in the bacterial flora of the gut due to long periods of drug therapy or several years on a poor diet, patients may find their constipation is relieved if they also avoid refined carbohydrates, such as sugar and foods containing sugar and white flour.

They should also realise that many drugs have a constipating effect.

Opiates, iron tablets, certain antidepressants and antacids can all reduce the natural movements of the gut.

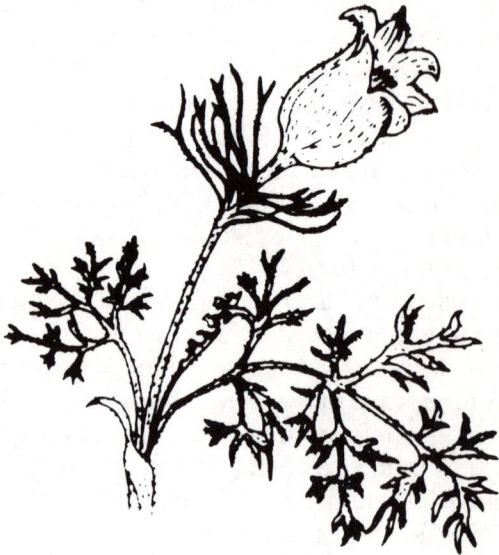

Chapter 4

Dealing with Diarrhoea

Diarrhoea, perhaps several times a day, accompanied by flatulence, is one of the most distressing aspects of the irritable bowel syndrome.

A complaint of diarrhoea must always be regarded as an important symptom until proved otherwise, because it can also occur with more serious conditions, such as coeliac disease, ulcerative colitis, Crohn's disease, or with tumours of the colon or endocrine system.

I have on my files the case of a professional man in his thirties, who first complained of abdominal pain and bowel dysfunction when he was only seven years old. He was taken to see his doctor, who prescribed medicine, but never requested any proper investigation by a consultant.

The pain continued intermittently throughout his life and eventually he was told he was suffering from irritable bowel syndrome.

However, no medication was ever successful in clearing it up. The pain continued and the frequency of his bowel motions, now very watery, gradually increased to between 14 and 16 a day.

He also began passing blood — another serious sign. At this stage he was referred to a gastroenterologist who, on investigating the bowel discovered it was so ulcerated that it might have to be removed. The man was given analgesics, oral prednisolone and steroid suppositories.

At this point he became so upset and disillusioned with his medical treatment which had never attempted to discover the cause of his suffering, but only to treat the symptoms, that he decided to seek alternative advice.

The herbal and naturopathic approach to the treatment of inflammatory bowel disease is outside the scope of this book, but the case is included in order to highlight the consequences of improper diagnosis.

Unfortunately, it is not unusual for inflammatory bowel disease to be overlooked by busy physicians.

It should be a rule not to continue to treat chronic diarrhoea for more than a fortnight without an appropriate investigation being undertaken.

Of course, one person's idea of what constitutes diarrhoea can be totally different to somebody else's. Some people think they have diarrhoea if their stools become softer than usual and they pass wind at the same time.

As a symptom of irritable bowel syndrome, diarrhoea rarely occurs during the night. It has been found that people who do suffer spontaneous night attacks of diarrhoea are much more likely to be suffering from an organic, rather than a functional disease.

Many people suffer from diarrhoea because of laxative abuse. They believe it is a good thing to have a 'proper clearout' every day. But only gentle herbal laxatives should be used when necessary: they should not become a habit. It is far better to improve the diet rather than resort to chronic laxative abuse.

The use of unprocessed wheatbran — two tablespoonfuls sprinkled over a breakfast cereal — may be all that is necessary to alleviate irritable bowel in both those who are mainly plagued with constipation and in those who mainly suffer diarrhoea.

However, for reasons given in other parts of this book it does not suit everybody. Indeed, and this might surprise many physicians who feel they are experts in the matter, Captain Peter Cleave, a surgeon in the Royal Navy, who first put forward the fibre theory of disease, did not consider that bran was the treatment of choice for irritable bowel.

It is sufficient to say that the medical profession's understanding of Cleave's fibre theory is still wholly inadequate.

After first resisting the idea that fibre was an important part of our food they now prescribe it on its own as though it were a medicine, or drug, instead of part of a healthy, wholefood regime.

As a medical journalist I interviewed the naval surgeon, Peter Cleave, several times at his home near the south coast in the 1970s after he had written his book *The Saccharine Disease*, for which he should have received a Nobel prize.

He told me quite clearly that he disagreed with those who believed that the successful treatment of irritable colon lay with unprocessed bran on its own, although he thought a wholemeal loaf was an excellent food to recommend.

No, his experience was that white, refined sugar was the main culprit, and that it should be replaced in the diet by all forms of raw and dried fruit (but not tinned fruit) and by fresh vegetables.

The basis of his argument was that many of man's diseases in the West were the result of the food manufacturers stripping fibre out of our food, which leads inevitably to the over-consumption of refined carbohydrates, that is white flour, white sugar, white rice and white pasta. He was, however, a strong advocate of unprocessed bran for the treatment of constipation.

HERBS

A number of herbs are invaluable in treating diarrhoea and these will be found in the herb list section of this book.

But a good first choice for simple diarrhoea would be Meadowsweet, also known as Queen of the Meadow, which was indeed a favourite herb with Queen Elizabeth the First, not in her case for the treatment of diarrhoea, but as an aromatic herb, the flowers of which were used as a bedroom freshener.

An infusion of this common wild plant taken in doses of two fluid ounces slows the motility of the intestinal canal and thus helps to regulate the bowel motions. It is not unpleasant to take and can also be given in smaller doses to children with bowel irregularity.

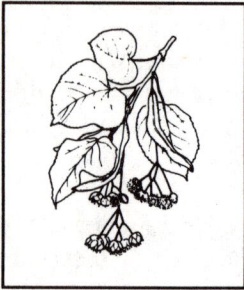

Lime Flowers

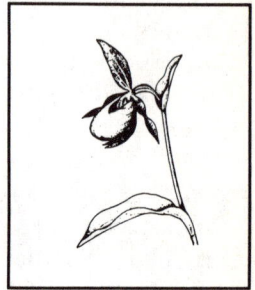

Lady's slipper

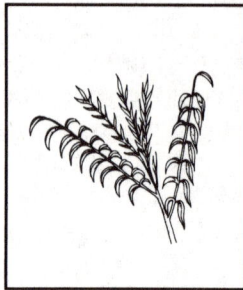

Liquorice

Chapter 5

Wind and Gas —
Where does it come from?

Medical people call it flatulence or gas, whereas most non-medical people refer to it as 'passing or breaking wind' — 'farting' (if passed downwards) and 'belching' if released upwards from the stomach.

Where does all this gas come from? Most of it is produced by bacteria which feed on undigested particles of food that travel along the gastrointestinal tract. Much of the undigested food, or residue, is made of fibre, which stimulates the bowel to work — a snake-like movement known as peristalsis.

As the particles move along, the bacteria which normally inhabit the healthy bowel feed on the fibre and then produce gas and other waste products. The gas is, therefore, a bacterial excrement, but the whole process is described as fermentation. It is similar to the yeast fermentation which home brewers rely on to produce alcohol.

The residue from natural foods tends to promote the survival of friendly bacteria which aid in the production of vitamins.

Residue from foods which are unhealthy, such as refined sugars, cause the bowel to over-populate itself with unfriendly bacteria. We then say that the 'bowel flora' is out of balance. Drugs, such as antibiotics, also wipe out friendly bacteria, and encourage the reproduction of yeast organisms in the bowel, such as *Candida albicans*.

Bacteria can produce larger amounts of gas from some food fibres than from others. It is well known, for example,

31

that baked beans cause a lot of gas to be formed.

The speed at which the residue travels through the colon is also important in flatulence. The slower the transit time through the intestinal tract the longer the bacteria have to feed and, consequently, the greater the gas produced.

Sufferers from irritable bowel who produce a lot of gas should first examine their diet to see if they are including too many flatulent foods. These are usually foods with hard fibres, such as beans, onions and peppers. These foods, because they are tough as well as indigestible, are also the ones most likely to cause bowel pain.

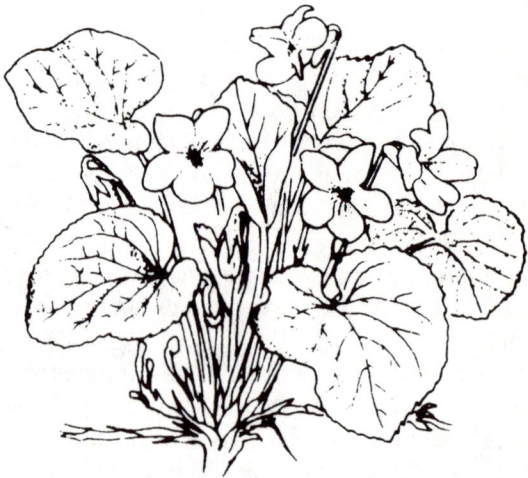

Chapter 6

The Allergic Bowel

Two-thirds of all cases of irritable bowel are due to food intolerance. This has been proven in clinical trials which showed that patients become free of symptoms if they follow diets which exclude common food allergens.

In many cases, people enjoy the foods or drinks that they are sensitive to and may find it difficult to give them up.

The most common foods found to cause IBS are milk, wheat, eggs, citrus fruit, chocolate and onions. Tea and coffee drinking are also high on the list.

Other foods found to cause bowel symptoms are potatoes, bananas, peanuts, brassicas and corn.

A complicating factor is that most people with "allergic bowel" react to more than one food, so that just leaving out one suspected item of food at a time may not solve the problem.

Without going as far as a complete fast, the best approach is to exclude from the diet as many as possible of the common causes of food allergy. I would always exclude milk, chocolate, wheat products, including bread and cereals, and tea and coffee for a trial period.

This kind of dieting is easy to do at home. But more complex exclusion diets need to be done under supervision to make sure that a nutritionally balanced menu is being followed and to deal with any side effects that may be experienced.

It is not unusual, for example, to develop a headache in the first day or two while on a restricted diet. The fact that wheat goes into a commercially manufactured food may also be overlooked. I have found that milk is more often associated with diarrhoea than with constipation and wheat with flatulence.

It can be seen from this that if IBS is due to a reaction to wheat, then not much good will come from adding bran or a wheat cereal to the diet to try to increase the fibre content.

It is suggested therefore, that the possibility of food intolerance or allergy is not investigated until after a reasonable period of experimenting with a high fibre diet.

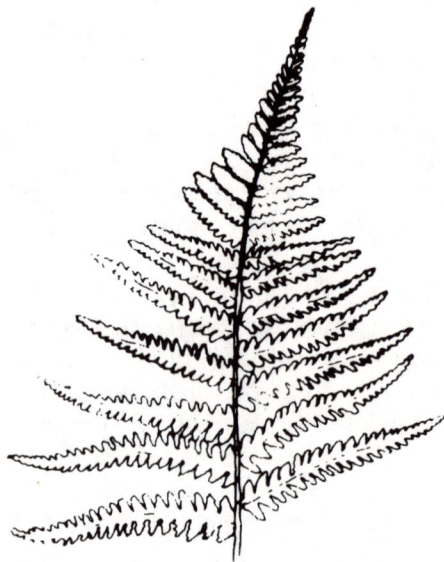

Chapter 7

The Fibre Factor

Irritable bowel syndrome in which the chief symptoms are constipation accompanied by abdominal pain is often the result of years spent on a fibre-depleted diet.

This type of IBS will generally respond to simple dietary modification which entails the addition of more fibre to the diet and a reduction in refined carbohydrates. Emollient herbal medicines, such as decoction of Marshmallow root, which soothe the internal surface of the colon, are also indicated.

Although unprocessed bran is considered by some to be laxative, it is in fact a stool-bulking agent. It turns small hard pellety stools into large soft ones which are more easily passed and which move through the intestinal canal at a respectable rate instead of being held up for days in a colon that has lost its tone.

There is as yet no drug or manufactured product available which can equal the use of unprocessed bran as a stool-bulking agent. The stool is largely made up of water and stool-bulking agents work by absorbing water.

The secret of the success of bran is that it is capable of holding about five times its own weight in water. Coarse bran can hold 2½ times the amount held by fine bran.

With different types of fibre there are other factors that may need to be taken into account.

For example, ispaghula husk increases stool bulk but may raise pressure inside the colon, which is undesirable as it can produce more pain. Fruit and vegetables are generally rich in fibre but may well act by increasing the bacterial population in the bowel.

A number of vegetables and fruit can be compared to bran for their water-holding and therefore their stool-bulking properties. Carrots, for example, hold twice their own weight, closely followed by apples, brussels sprouts and oatmeal.

Aubergines, spring cabbage, corn, oranges and pears hold little more than their own weight.

In the third division, as far as fibre is concerned, the list continues down through green beans, lettuce, cabbage, peas, onion, celery, cucumber, broad beans, tomato, cauliflower, banana, rhubarb, old potato, new potato, to turnip, which holds just under half its own weight.

As well as influencing stool size and weight, fibre affects the rate that food empties from the stomach and the absorption of nutrients through the bowel wall into the blood.

Different types of dietary fibre, such as cellulose, pectin and mucilage, act differently in the body. Cellulose, very rich in bran, boosts stool weight, and is mostly excreted in the faeces, although some is fermented (or digested) by bacteria in the colon to produce useful products, at least one of which is considered to be anti-cancerous.

Pectin, found in all plants, but notably in fruit peel and rind, is able to lower serum cholesterol levels, and mucilage found in seeds and specific medicinal herbs, is soothing to the internal surface of the colon.

Chapter 8

Controlling Candida

Although it has been denied several times in medical journals by those who should know better there is undoubtedly an epidemic of candidiasis in the UK.

This condition, due to an overgrowth of a yeast organism, *Candida albicans*, in the bowel, is commonly known as thrush. It is easily recognised when it occurs in the mouth or vagina, but often overlooked when it affects the bowel.

However, one of the major signs of candida overgrowth is an irritable colon. The condition includes all the usual IBS symptoms — alternating diarrhoea and constipation, flatulence, abdominal distension and pain, and rectal irritation or itching.

There have always been cases of candidiasis, but the current epidemic is without any doubt due to the overuse of antibiotics and steroid drugs, including the oral contraceptive pill. At one time the antifungal drugs used to treat candidiasis was a Cinderella industry. But with the advent of the drugs mentioned above it has become a multi-million pound one. This in itself is enough proof that an epidemic exists.

These drugs alter the bowel environment, either by killing off organisms detrimental to *Candida albicans*, or by altering the acid-alkaline balance in favour of the organism. Candida, which is a normal inhabitant of the bowel, does no harm when its population level in the body is kept under control naturally, but when conditions change so that reproduction of the organism is encouraged, it begins to spread — and can do so throughout the body.

Other factors which encourage candida to multiply include the overuse of refined carbohydrates in the diet, such as white sugar, white flour, white rice and white pasta, and foods which benefit a yeast environment such as bread, alcohol, and other yeast products. A deficiency of the digestive juices which tend to inhibit candida reproduction may also be a cause.

It is recommended that if candidiasis is suspected as being the cause of irritable bowel syndrome, professional help should be sought, and that a more specialist book on the subject be read.

However, certain self-help measures can be taken. The first is to add live yoghurt to the diet on a daily basis as this contains bacteria which control *Candida albicans* in the bowel. If yoghurt is not an acceptable food then the bacteria, Lactobacillus acidophilus, can be taken in capsule form obtainable from health stores.

Second, take plenty of garlic, garlic oil in capsules, or pressed garlic in tablet form. Garlic is a potent antifungal agent and suppresses the growth of candida.

Other plant remedies that are effective against candida include goldenseal, rosemary, wild chamomile, lemon balm, cinnamon and ginger.

Chapter 9

Milk —
the Good and the Bad

There are many arguments for and against the use of milk as a food for humans. It is, like other dairy products, an easily accessible source of first-class protein. When I was at school we were given a bottle of milk every day, because it was said to build healthy children. The calcium it contains is essential for strong bones and teeth, and a glass of milk at night helps to ensure restful sleep.

Many nature cure clinics and naturopathic doctors have in the past used milk diets as a universal treatment for all kinds of disease.

However, they were more inclined to use raw un-pasteurised cow's milk and to give detailed instructions on how to drink it.

They found that anyone suffering from any form of gastrointestinal disorder would usually improve significantly after a few days on a milk diet as it would assist the stomach and intestines to regain their normal tone. The rest from other foods would also be of undoubted benefit.

The patient was directed to take the milk in place of all other foods and, if wished, could use up to a quart at a time. The method of choice, however, was to drink small quantities at frequent intervals — say, every hour, consuming a total of about three quarts a day.

In addition the patient was advised to take one or more teaspoonsful of fruit juice — lemon, orange, or grapefruit — just before taking each glass of milk. It was believed that this aided the digestion of the milk by emulsifying the fat and prevented biliousness. It enabled more people to follow the milk diet than one would otherwise expect.

A modified method was to drink a glass of milk every 15 minutes until a quart had been taken and to eat some of the fruits mentioned along with it.

Patients on a milk diet were told not to simply swallow the milk down, but to masticate it as if it were a solid food by moving it around the mouth and mixing it with the saliva. Unless this was done large curds were likely to form in the stomach which the gastric juices were unable to penetrate and, therefore, insufficient nutrients would be extracted.

Milk, it was pointed out, was not as easily digested as popularly believed and took much the same time as for meat.

It was a rule that milk should never be taken with an ordinary meal containing meat or fish as this formed one of the most incompatible of food mixtures, an observation which, incidentally, had been made centuries earlier.

Perhaps this goes some way to explaining why other naturopaths and herbalists believed that cow's milk was not suitable for human consumption. Drinking milk, they said, led to biliousness, coated tongue and headache — typical symptoms of auto-intoxication. The argument as to whether milk should be taken raw or pasteurised still rages on. Certainly, milk from unhealthy animals cannot be made nutritious by pasteurising it and the law seems to be that raw milk cannot be sold by farmers unless it comes from disease free cows.

It is claimed by those who sell raw milk that it does not, for example, increase cholesterol levels in the blood because it contains anti-cholesterol compounds which, together with other valuable components, are destroyed in the pasteurising process.

I will not get involved in the vegan argument that

drinking milk is immoral, but would agree with the vegans that there are alternatives to cow's milk from plant sources which are nutritionally adequate.

And for people who are intolerant to milk, for one reason or another, plant milks are a suitable replacement as well as adding variety to the diet.

I was unable to drink pasteurised cow's milk at school for very long, because it was found that it "did not agree with me". It created mucous and catarrh, which made me feel ill, and caused me to cough at night, so I was "excused milk" by the teacher. I still never drink a glass of milk on its own and never put it on cereal. A dash of milk in other dishes does not seem to affect me unduly.

LACTOSE INTOLERANCE

As I mentioned briefly in Chapter 1 at least 10 per cent of cases of "irritable bowel" are due to milk intolerance.

Surprisingly, most people in the world are intolerant to milk, and for many people, including a number of babies, it is positively harmful. In the case of babies it makes no difference whether the milk is of animal or human origin.

The reason is that they are unable to digest lactose, the milk sugar, because the cells lining their intestines fail to produce lactase, an enzyme that breaks the lactose down into glucose and galactose. Unless it is broken down, the lactose cannot be absorbed from the intestine into the blood.

If they drink milk they will develop a number of symptoms, including nausea or vomiting, abdominal distension, or bloating, and flatulence. The stools tend to be watery and acidic, causing sore buttocks — even being abrasive enough to remove the skin — or the stools become bulky and loose.

The severity of the symptoms varies according to the age of the patient and the degree of lactase deficiency. In mild cases the person may complain only of gas and stools that are "a bit loose" and may never consider that what is normal for them is actually due to lactase deficiency.

There are a number of reasons why people become lactase deficient. The commonest reason is that milk, while being a natural food for babies and young children, is not so natural for older children and adults. As we grow older our ability to produce lactase is not so necessary.

However, it appears that most people belonging to white races, probably because they continue to use milk extensively in their diets, continue to produce lactase and are able to digest lactose for most of their lives, while most people of other races, including black Africans, Eskimos, Arabs, American Indians and Australian Aborigines, show a decline in intestinal lactase activity after the age of two — the age at which the "milk teeth" have been produced, and after which the need for milk is not so important.

With inter-racial marriage down the centuries there has been some mixing of lactase and non-lactase populations and there is no longer such a clear dividing line between the groups.

Another major cause of lactose intolerance results from damage to the intestinal lining due to coeliac disease or to gastroenteritis. Anyone who has suffered a severe attack of gastroenteritis, followed by irritable bowel should suspect lactase deficiency.

Some people are born with lactose intolerance. Although the intestinal lining is normal, there is an absence of lactase production. This is usually diagnosed soon after birth as the baby fails to thrive on breast milk, or milk formulas, and needs to be given a lactose-free feed.

Babies who are born prematurely may not have developed their lactase production sufficiently to digest lactose and they too will suffer diarrhoea and vomiting unless given a lactose-free feed. However, after a few weeks they start producing their own lactase and are then able to begin digesting milk properly.

The most common, but sometimes baffling cause of lactose intolerance in babies, is when it follows an attack of gastroenteritis — baffling because the symptoms recur immediately feeding is restarted and when it seems that the baby is over the initial attack.

Correct diagnosis by a paediatrician is obviously vitally important at this stage as lactose-free feeds can lead to a rapid improvement, and may be needed for only a few weeks.

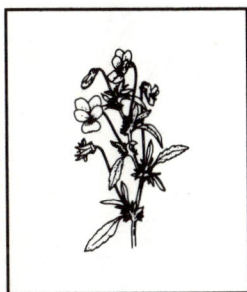

Heartease

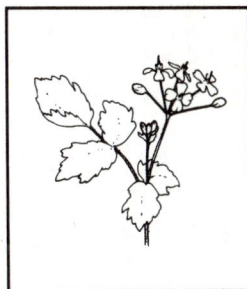

Celandine

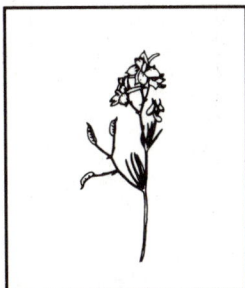

Larkspur

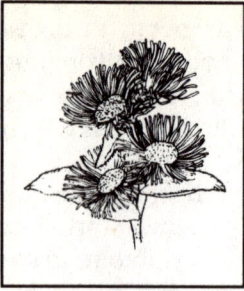

Elecampane

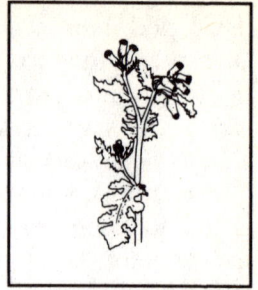

Groundsel

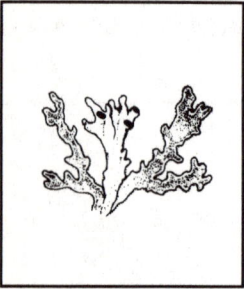

Iceland Moss

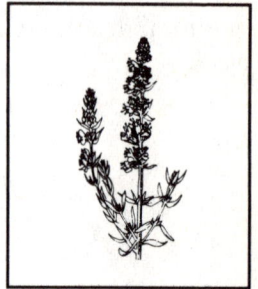

Hyssop

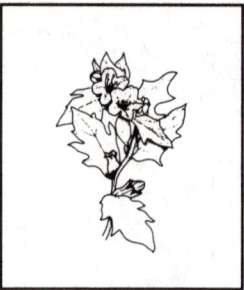

Horehound

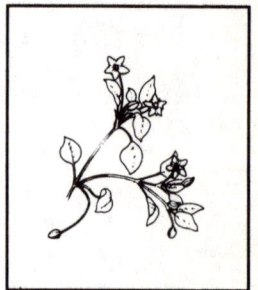

Chickweed

Chapter 10

Laxative Abuse

According to the medical newspaper, GP*, hundreds of people undergo expensive but unnecessary hospital investigations for chronic diarrhoea.

The investigations, including laparotomy, are unnecessary because the patients are simply abusing laxatives. They could have been diagnosed quite cheaply by screening for laxative drugs in their urine.

Doctors at the Royal Infirmary, Glasgow, say that about 75 per cent of patients with laxative-induced diarrhoea are overlooked by family doctors, largely due to poor clinical awareness. They are often diagnosed as suffering from irritable bowel syndrome.

One patient had more that £10,000 worth of investigations before it was discovered that they were surreptitiously self-medicating with laxatives.

*GP, April 3rd, 1992.

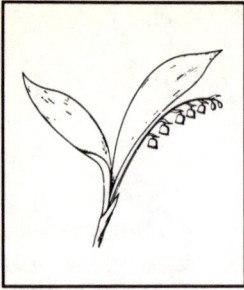

Lily of the Valley

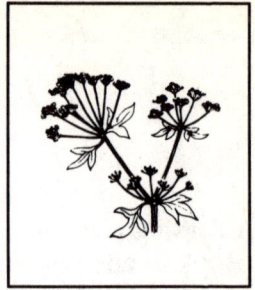

Celery

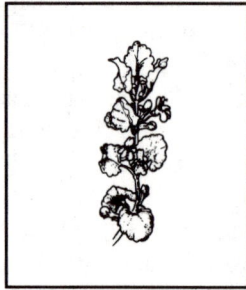

Ground Ivy

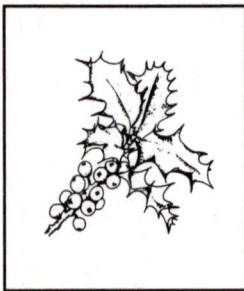

Holly

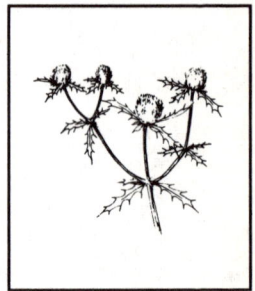

Eryngo

Chapter 11

Drugs that affect the Bowel

It is most likely that the sufferer from symptoms of an irritable bowel will have consulted their family doctor, or have been referred to a gastroenterologist. And the chances are that in addition to some cursory advice to eat more bran they will have received one or more medicines.

There is a heavy demand in Britain and Europe for stomach and bowel remedies — and even more so in the United States.

It must be a commentary on the dietary habits of people in the Western world that there are so many diseased digestive systems, painful stomachs, and irritable bowels.

Manufacturing medicines for prescription and over-the-counter sales is a multi-million pound industry — and yet much of this would be entirely unnecessary, if only a sensible approach to eating was taken as outlined in this book.

In treating gastrointestinal disease doctors have a wide range of drugs to choose from, including antacids, antiflatulents, reflux suppressants and antispasmodics, bulking agents, antidiarrhoeals, and not least tranquillisers.

The routine prescription of drugs has been questioned as there is little good research to substantiate their efficacy.

An important review of 43 clinical trials of drugs prescribed for irritable bowel syndrome published in the medical journal *Gastroenterology* in 1988 concluded that there was no convincing evidence that any drug prescribed for IBS was effective.

47

The author did concede that individual symptoms such as diarrhoea could be alleviated with a specific drug but stressed that there was no drug available to treat irritable bowel syndrome in its entirety. However, there are a whole range of other drugs, including non-steroidal anti-inflammatory agents, prescribed on a daily basis by doctors, that actually cause digestive problems.

This chapter outlines some of the drugs prescribed by doctors, together with some of the side effects and adverse reactions associated with them. The information has not been given to alarm anyone who may be taking any of these drugs, but to make them aware of their possible effects.

However, it should be emphasised that people react differently to drugs and that not everyone will, necessarily, suffer side-effects.

Unfortunately, many doctors fail to explain to their patients that gastrointestinal side effects can be expected from a particular drug, or course of treatment, and this may cause great distress. This is often due to a failure to communicate since pharmaceutical companies usually advise doctors of the side effects reported during the clinical trials of their medicines.

There is often more than one proprietary brand of a drug, particularly where the patient for the original drug has expired. Brand names are given in brackets.

Note: Do not stop taking any medication prescribed by your doctor without prior consultation and do not take herbal medicines along with medicines from your doctor without proper advice.

BENORYLATE
(Benoral)
Indications: Rheumatoid arthritis, osteoarthritis and other painful musculoskeletal conditions.

Possible side effects: Gastrointestinal upset.

CISAPRIDE
(Alimix, Prepulsid)
Indications: Symptoms associated with acid reflux.

Possible side effects: Diarrhoea, abdominal cramps and intestinal rumblings.

DIFLUNISAL
(Dolobid)
Indications: Rheumatoid arthritis and osteoarthritis

Possible side effects: Gastric disturbance, stomach pains, indigestion, diarrhoea.

FENOPROFEN
(Fenopron)
Indications: Rheumatoid arthritis, osteoarthritis, ankylosing spondylitis.

Possible side effects: Gastric disturbances, allergies, liver disorders.

FLURBIPROFEN
(Froben)
Indications: Rheumatoid arthritis, osteoarthritis, ankylosing spondylitis.

**Possible
side effects:**   Gastric upset.

IBUPROFEN
(Brufen)
Indications: Adult and juvenile rheumatoid
                                    arthritis, osteoarthritis,
                                    ankylosing spondylitis, soft tissue
                                    injuries.

**Possible
side effects:**   Gastric bleeding, indigestion.

INDOMETHACIN
(Indocid)
Indications: Acute gout, rheumatoid arthritis,
                                    osteoarthritis, ankylosing
                                    spondylitis, acute joint disorders.

**Possible
side effects:**   Gastric bleeding.

KETOPROFEN
(Orudis)
(Oruvail)
Indications: Rheumatoid arthritis,
                                    osteoarthrosis, ankylosing
                                    spondylitis, acute joint disease,
                                    acute gout.

**Possible
side effects:**   Gastric upsets.

MEFENAMIC ACID
(Ponstan Forte)
Indications: Painful rheumatoid arthritis and
                                    Still's disease, and osteoarthrosis.

**Possible
side effects:**   Diarrhoea.

NAPROXEN
(Naprosyn)
Indications: Acute gout, ankylosing
spondylitis, rheumatoid arthritis,
osteoarthritis.

Possible   Gastric disturbances.
side effects:

PREDNISONE
(Decortisyl)
Indications: Rheumatic conditions
Possible   Peptic ulceration.
side effects:

PREDNISOLONE
(Deltacortril)
(Prednesol)
Indications: Rheumatic conditions
Possible   Similar to prednisone.
side effects:

SODIUM AUROTHIOMALATE
(Myocrisin)
Indications: Rheumatoid arthritis.

Possible   This drug (a gold salt) is given
side effects: by injection. The treatment can
induce diarrhoea, metallic taste.

SULINDAC
(Clinoril)
Indications: Acute gout and joint conditions,
ankylosing spondylitis,
rheumatoid arthritis,
osteoarthrosis.

| **Possible side effects:** | Stomach pain, indigestion, bitter taste in mouth. |

STERCULIA/ALVERINE CITRATE
(Alvercol)

| **Indications:** | Irritable bowel syndrome. |
| **Possible side effects:** | Occasional mild distension. |

SUCRALFATE
(Antepsin)

| **Indications:** | Duodenal and peptic ulcers. |
| **Possible side effects:** | Gastrointestinal upset, constipation, diarrhoea. |

MEPENZOLATE BROMIDE
(Cantil)

| **Indications::** | Spasm of large bowel |
| **Possible side effects:** | Constipation, nausea, difficulty in swallowing. |

MISOPROSTOL
(Cytotec)

| **Indications:** | Stomach and duodenal ulcers. |
| **Possible side effects:** | Diarrhoea, abdominal pain, gastrointestinal upset. |

CIMETIDINE
(Dyspamet, Tagamet)

| **Indications::** | Dyspepsia due to acidity |
| **Possible side effects:** | Diarrhoea. |

OMEPRAZOLE
(Losec)

Indications: Peptic ulcers, acid reflux

Possible side effects: Diarrhoea, constipation, nausea.

METOCLOPRAMIDE
(Maxolon)

Indications: Flatulence, indigestion, heartburn

Possible side effects: Diarrhoea.

FAMOTIDINE
(Pepcid PM)

Indications: Duodenal and stomach ulcers

Possible side effects: Diarrhoea, constipation, nausea, gastrointestinal discomfort, loss of appetite.

PIPENZOLATE BROMIDE
(Piptal)

Indications: Excessive intestinal motility

Possible side effects: Constipation, nausea, dry mouth.

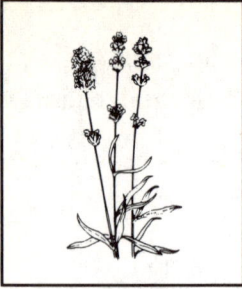

Lavender

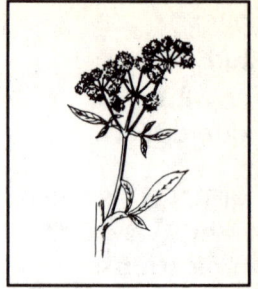

Lovage

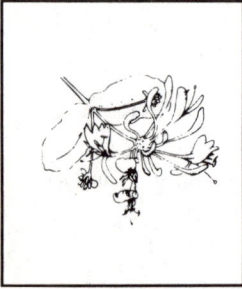

Honeysuckle

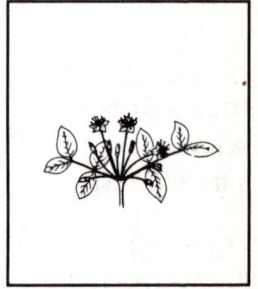

Guaiacum

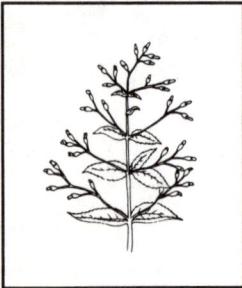

Lobelia

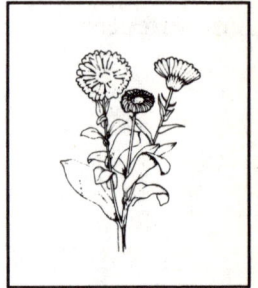

Marigold

Chapter 12

Herbal Preparations

Although herbal products are widely available from health stores and other retail outlets, traditional preparations made at home are in many ways superior. Most medical herbalists would agree that, where the medicinal properties of a herb are soluble in water, infusions and decoctions are an effective way to take them.

Caution with all medicines, including herbs, is advised during pregnancy. While most are safe, a few are contraindicated and, therefore, they should be taken at this time only under supervision of a qualified practitioner. The same caution applies to the treatment of babies and young children.

INFUSIONS
Infusions, also known as teas or tisanes, are usually made with the softer parts of the plant, such as the flowers or leaves. Chop these finely and place about an ounce in a jug, preferably one with a close fitting lid. Pour a pint (20 fluid ounces) of boiling water on to the herb and cover the jug. Infuse the herb for 10 to 15 minutes, stirring occasionally. When ready strain off the tea. The usual dose range is from ½ to two fluid ounces three times a day. If the medicine is to be taken on a long-term basis half an ounce to one pint of water is usually recommended.

DECOCTIONS
Decoctions are more suitable for the harder parts of the plant, such as the bark, roots and berries. To every ounce of

the plant material, which is best ground down into a rough powder, or finely chopped, pour on 1½ pints (30 fluid ounces) of cold water, cover and allow to stand overnight. Then bring to the boil and simmer for 20 minutes, or until there is a pint (20 fluid ounces) of water left. Strain and drink from ½ to 2 fluid ounces two or three times a day.

Infusions and decoctions can also be made in a coffee percolator.

TINCTURES
These are used when the medicinal properties are either destroyed by heat, or not sufficiently soluble in water. The herb is steeped (macerated) in a mixture (known as the menstruum) of alcohol and cold water – usually a minimum of 20 per cent pure alcohol – for at least two weeks before being pressed out and filtered ready for use. The tinctures prescribed by medical herbalists are made with pure alcohol for which a government licence is necessary. They may also undergo the process of maceration and filtration several times in order to strengthen the tincture and to reduce the final alcohol content to a minimum.

For home use tinctures can be made with brandy, but this is rather an expensive process. However, the preparation is much stronger than a simple infusion or decoction, the ratio being 1:5 – one ounce of the herb to five fluid ounces of menstruum. Most tinctures need a 25 per cent proportion of alcohol to water. Dosage ranges from 10–40 drops (¼ml–2ml), except for the more potent remedies. The advantage of tinctures is that they are more convenient to use and they keep well.

Some herbalists, including myself, prefer tinctures made in the ratio of 1:3 – one ounce of herb to three ounces of menstruum. On filtration the amount of tincture recovered is made equal to the original amount, that is three ounces, by making up the amount with further menstruum, or by re-maceration.

FLUID EXTRACTS
Strong tinctures, or fluid extracts, can be made by reducing the final amount recovered. This is achieved by evaporation on a very low heat for several hours using a water bath, or double saucepan. An official fluid extract is one that contains the equivalent of one ounce of herb to every fluid ounce of extract (a ratio of 1:1) and contains an adequate amount of alcohol to preserve it.

LOTIONS
Medicinal preparations such as lotions, mouth washes, gargles and douches can be made from infusions. They are best filtered after straining off the herb.

ESSENTIAL OILS
Pure oils extracted from plants are extremely potent – and toxic in overdose – and should not be taken internally without adequate knowledge of the individual remedy. Many of them tend to be antifungal and antibiotic in action. One drop of the oil, shaken in water, at most forms a single dose. One drop of peppermint oil dropped on to the tongue is so strong it makes the eyes water. The potency of essential oils can be seen from the effect of just adding a few drops into bath water. Prescribed correctly, plant oils are a useful addition to the herbal dispensary. Appropriate remedies can be diluted one part in a hundred parts of water and used in douches.

INFUSED OILS
These are quite different from essential oils. Herbs, such as Calendula and Comfrey are steeped in a bland oil, such as olive oil, in a warm place – traditionally in the sun – for at

least two weeks so that the medicinal properties are infused into the oil. They are then strained ready for use. Infused oils are excellent for external use and, therefore, the strength may vary. One can keep repeating the infusion process by adding more herb to the oil and setting aside for a further time. A practitioner would use an infused oil of comfrey, for example, for deep massage of the abdomen to improve circulation and to help remove toxic waste from the colon.

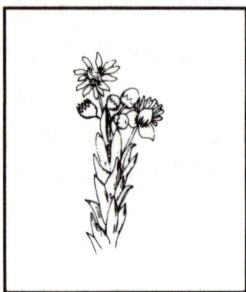

Houseleek

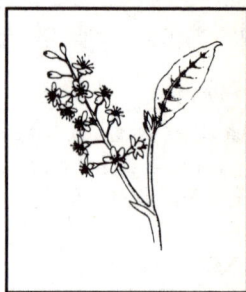

Cherry Laurel

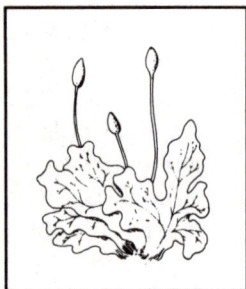

Liverwort (English)

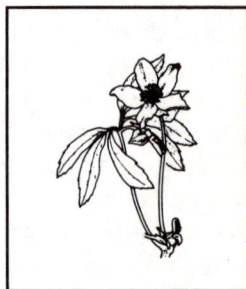

Hellebore, Black

Chapter 13

Selected Herbs

MEADOWSWEET

This is a favourite herb of professional herbal practitioners for treating gastrointestinal disorders. Meadowsweet, known to herbalists as *Spiraea ulmaria,* is a gentle, healing herb, yet is a very effective remedy for the diarrhoea associated with irritable bowel syndrome and for simple attacks of diarrhoea, particularly in children.

The 17th century herbalist Nicholas Culpeper observed that it was an excellent medicine in fevers "attended with purgings" and useful "in all fluxes".

It is known by one or two other common names, including Queen of the Meadow and Lady of the Meadow. It grows as its name suggests in moist meadows and in clearings in woodland, but it also seems happy by riversides. There is, for example, quite a lot of meadowsweet growing by the river Thames at Reading.

As meadowsweet has been used in beer-making, one often finds it growing on fields near to village inns, because the seeds have travelled with the lorries delivering the barrels and have then blown into the fields and seeded themselves.

The white flowers, which resemble the garden varieties of Spiraea, appear in early summer and are pleasantly fragrant. They were once strewn on the floors of houses to clear the rooms of bad smells.

An infusion is made by steeping one ounce of the fresh flowers in about one pint (20fl.oz) of boiling water. It is then strained and taken in wineglassful doses (2fl.oz). Tinctures are prescribed by herbalists.

In addition to easing diarrhoea, because of its mild astringency, it is a useful remedy for acid eructations from the stomach and for indigestion — meadowsweet has become known as the herbal bicarbonate of soda. Used over a period of time it will help to normalise production of gastric juices. It combines well with liquorice, which is soothing to the stomach and intestinal canal, and dandelion root, which helps digestion by stimulating liver and gall bladder function and increasing the production of bile.

For acid conditions simmer half an ounce each of liquorice and dandelion root first, as if making a decoction, in 1½ pints of water and then remove from the heat and add ½oz of meadowsweet and a quarter-ounce of peppermint herb. Infuse until cool and then add honey to taste. Take in doses of from two teaspoonfuls to 2fl.oz. three or four times a day, according to age.

MARSHMALLOW

The herb that soothes. Marshmallow is mainly used for its emollient effect when the gastrointestinal canal is irritated or inflamed. Its official name, *Althaea officinalis*, means to cure, while mallow means to soften.

Like meadowsweet it thrives in damp meadows and on the banks of the river. It was always grown in gardens in former times because of its medicinal properties and it is thought that the plant was introduced into Britain by the Romans. As all of the medicinal properties are soluble in water it is an ideal remedy for domestic use either as an infusion of the leaves or a decoction of the root.

To make an infusion use 1oz of the leaves, picked from the plant just as the flowers are coming into bloom. Add them to one pint of boiling water and allow to cool. Strain and add honey or orange juice. The dose is 2fl.oz. three or four times a day. This is an ideal remedy for the elderly suffering from chronic inflammatory conditions of the colon. It is used extensively for colitis and gastritis.

Marshmallow root, which is available dried, produces a mucilage when boiled which is healing to the colon. It can replace the mucous lost from the surface of the intestinal canal. It can be combined with slippery elm, another important demulcent, and chickweed, an effective anti-inflammatory agent.

Simmer half an ounce of each in two pints of water until the total is reduced to 1½pts. Strain and add honey to taste. Doses of 2fl.oz. can be taken three or four times a day.

SLIPPERY ELM

When one considers that Slippery Elm is one of the most useful of all medicinal plants, it is surprising that so many people have never heard of it.

A teaspoonful of powdered bark is placed in a jug, and a pint of boiling water slowly poured on to it, mixing constantly as if making a delicate sauce. If the mixture becomes lumpy strain it before use. It can be flavoured with a pinch of powdered nutmeg or cinnamon.

Not only is the bark healing and soothing, but it is also nutritional and is known as slippery elm food. It can be given to babies and invalids and will be nourishing when other foods cannot be taken.

In serious diseases when ordinary food cannot be given orally it has been injected into the bowel to provide a valuable source of nutrition.

Countless cases of irritated colon, diarrhoea and dysentery, have been cured with its use. It has a reputation as a leading healing agent in peptic and duodenal ulcers and in intestinal inflammation, including mucous colitis and gastroenteritis, both in children and adults.

An official mucilage is made by simmering six grams of the bark in 100cc of water for one hour and then straining it.

In the traditional treatment of chronic diarrhoea, slippery elm powder is mixed with powdered bayberry bark and powdered scullcap – a teaspoonful of each – and infused in half a pint of boiling water for about 30 minutes. The mixture is strained and a teaspoonful of tincture of myrrh, a potent antiseptic, is added. It is then used as an injection direct into the bowel.

LIQUORICE

One of the oldest of medicinal herbs, and one of the more pleasant, there are few drugs to equal its ability to heal the damaged gastrointestinal mucosa.

It is added to herbal mixtures to improve their medicinal virtues and their taste. Its official name, *Glycyrrhiza glabra*, refers to its sweetness.

Liquorice, which has a feathery appearance, grows on sandy soils near water. The roots grow deep into the ground. It is used medicinally as a demulcent and is particularly soothing to the intestinal and respiratory tracts.

The infusion of 1oz of bruised root, with bark removed, in one pint of boiling water is used for internal ulcers and gastric catarrh. Drink a wineglassful three times a day. A strong decoction of the root will relieve constipation and can be given to children for this purpose.

Liquorice is contra-indicated in people who suffer from blood pressure as it tends to increase fluid retention.

Chapter 14

Herbs for the Bowel

Herbs have been used in the treatment of digestive disease throughout the ages. This section contains a description of remedies frequently prescribed by herbalists to alleviate the symptoms associated with irritable bowel syndrome and other important digestive disorders. A few herbal medicines may be available only on prescription from a medical herbalist.

Agrimony
AGRIMONIA EUPATORIA

Also know as	Church steeples
Where found	Throughout northern Europe
Appearance	A strong growing herb with green/grey leaves with soft hairs. Flowers are small and yellow on long slender spikes.
Part used	Herb
Therapeutic uses	A general tonic with astringent and diurectic properties. The dried leaves when infused are useful in treating simple diarrhoea and general intestinal debility, and to help prevent tissue wasting due to malabsorption. Agrimony also helps to clear skin eruptions, pimples and blotches.
Prepared as	Infusion, tincture.

Aniseed
PIMPINELLA ANISUM

Also know as	Anise
Where found	Grown in Southern Europe, North Africa, India and South America.
Appearance	White flowering garden herb with feathery leaves, growing to about 50cm high.
Part used	Seeds.
Therapeutic uses	A valuable carminative, useful in flatulence and colic.
Prepared as	Powder, infusion, tincture, essential oil.

Bayberry
MYRICA CERIFERA

Also known as	Candle Berry
Where found	United States
Appearance	Shrub up to 8ft high with shiny leaves and globular berries.
Part used	Bark.
Therapeutic uses	Stimulating and astringent; it improves circulation, and cleanses the stomach and bowels of catarrh. It has a positive effect on the circulatory system of the uterus and is a useful treatment for prolapse of that organ. Also for heavy periods, vaginitis, and simple vaginal discharge.
Prepared as	Powder, fluid extract, tincture, decoction, douche.

Black Cohosh
CIMICIFUGA RACEMOSA

Also known as — Squaw Root

Where found — United States and Canada

Appearance — A tall herbaceous plant with white feathery flowers.

Part used — Rhizome

Therapeutic uses — An antispasmodic, sedative, blood purifier and nervine. Used in small doses for children's diarrhoea. Large doses may cause nausea and vomiting. It is anti-flatulent.

Prepared as — Infusion, decoction, syrup, tincture.

Cardamom
ELETTARIA CARDAMOMUM

Also known as — Malabar Cardamom

Where found — Ceylon and India

Appearance — Forest plant with large smooth, dark green leaves and small yellowish flowers

Parts used — Fruits, seeds and oil

Therapeutic uses — An aromatic herb mainly used in the treatment of flatulence and other digestive problems. Cardamom is also reputed to be a sexual tonic. It is often used in aphrodisiac remedies.

Prepared as — Powder, liquid extract, tincture, essential oil.

Chamomile, wild
MATRICARIA CHAMOMILLA

Also known as	German chamomile
Where found	Corn fields in Europe
Appearance	Herb with small cushion-like flowers in profusion
Part used	Flowers
Therapeutic uses	A gastro-intestinal tonic and stimulating nervine, with carminative and antispasmodic properties. It reduces flatulence and abdominal distension and eases colicky pains and spasms in the colon. Continual daily use indicated in inflammatory and irritable bowel conditions. A chamomile poultice is healing to leg ulcers
Prepared as	Infusion, poultice, tincture.

Chamomile, common
ANTHEMIS NOBILIS

Also known as	Belgian chamomile
Where found	A favourite garden herb, abundant in France and Belgium, but widely cultivated.
Appearance	A herb resembling a large daisy with white flowers and yellow centres.
Parts used	Flowers and herb

Therapeutic uses	An antispasmodic indicated in stomach and intestinal disorders, including heartburn, simple indigestion, flatulence, colic, and for debilitated states of the colon. Also for simple diarrhoea in children. It is widely prescribed for nervous and hysterical conditions.
Prepared as	Infusion (chamomile tea), fluid extract, tincture.

Cinnamon
CINNAMOMUM ZEYLANICUM

Where found	A native plant of Ceylon
Appearance	A tree growing up to 30ft high in sandy soils.
Part used	Bark
Therapeutic uses	A carminative, aromatic, antiseptic, antifungal and stimulating astringent. It is very effective for treating vomiting and nausea, and will give relief in flatulence and diarrhoea.
Prepared as	Oil, medicinal water, tincture, powder.

Clary
SALVIA SCLAREA

Also known as	Christ's Eye and Clary Sage
Where found	Common garden plant

Appearance	Similar to common sage with blue or white flowers
Parts used	Herb, seeds and essential oil
Therapeutic uses	It is mainly used for digestive problems. It has antispasmodic properties which are useful in colic and painful menstruation. The old herbalists used it for ophthalmic conditions (clary eye = clear eye). Do not use this herb during pregnancy. The oil is intoxicating, which may have led to it being regarded as an aphrodisiac. It has been used as a sexual tonic in impotence and as a remedy for postnatal depression. Take under medical supervision.
Prepared as	infusion, mucilage and oil.

Cramp bark
VIBURNUM OPULUS

Also known as	Snowball tree, Guelder rose
Where found	Europe and the United States
Appearance	Strong-growing bush with white ball-shaped flowers.
Part used	Bark.
Therapeutic uses	Cramp bark, as its name suggests, is an antispasmodic. It is also an excellent nervine. It gives relief in gastrointestinal colic. As a nervine it is used in the treatment of spasms and convulsions.

Prepared as   Decoction, tincture.

Cranesbill
GERANIUM MACULTATUM

Also known as	Wild geranium
Where found	United States
Appearance	Shrubby small herb with blue flowers. The seed pod resembles a crane's bill.
Parts used	Herb and root
Therapeutic uses	Has styptic properties and is a tonic and astringent. Used in the treatment of ulcerated and mucous conditions of the gastrointestinal canal where there is diarrhoea, catarrhal discharge and bleeding. A useful treatment for piles.
Prepared as	Infusion of herb, decoction of root, powder, tincture.

Echinacea
ECHINACEA ANGUSTIFOLIA

Also known as	Cone flower
Where found	American prairies
Appearance	Herb of medium height
Part used	Rhizome

Therapeutic uses	Natural antibiotic, antiseptic and alterative. Helps to clear the blood of toxic material. Improves appetite and digestion. Used in ulcerative conditions of the stomach and duodenum to keep the tissues clean. Can be combined with goldenseal. Also used for boils and carbuncles.
Prepared as	Decoction, tincture.

Galangal
ALPINIA OFFICINARUM

Also known as	East Indian Root
Where found	China
Appearance	A tallish plant with long narrow leaves and white flowers with red veins.
Part used	Rhizome
Therapeutic uses	An excellent carminative, helping to relieve flatulence and reduce fermentation.
Prepared as	Decoction, powder, tincture.

Garlic
ALLIUM SATIVUM

Where found	Universally cultivated
Appearance	Similar to a shallot
Part used	Bulb

Therapeutic uses   For the treatment of dyspepsia
and flatulence. Garlic is a
powerful antiseptic and also
reduces cholesterol in the blood.

Prepared as   Powder, oil (in capsules), juice,
tablets and tincture.

Gentian
GENTIANA LUTEA

Also known as   Yellow Gentian

Where found   Alpine plant in Europe

Appearance   A hardy herbaceous perennial
bearing clusters of large orange-
yellow flowers.

Part used   Root

Therapeutic uses   One of the best gastrointestinal
tonics. It has a very bitter taste
even when greatly diluted. It
boosts appetite, aids digestion,
and is useful in cases of jaundice,
general debility and dyspepsia. It
is better to combine small doses
of the medicine with an aromatic
herb such as Cardamoms to help
camouflage the bitter taste.

Prepared as   Powder (use a quarter of a
teaspoonful infused in a cupful of
boiling water, sweetened with
honey), tincture.

Ginger
ZINGIBER OFFICINALE

Where found	West Indies and China
Appearance	About one metre high with glossy aromatic leaves.
Part used	Rhizome
Therapeutic uses	An excellent remedy for indigestion. Ginger is carminative — it reduces flatulence and distension and eases painful intestinal spasms. It also has stimulating and expectorant properties and is used in colds and chills.
Prepared as	Powder, syrup, tablets, tincture.

Goldenseal
HYDRASTIS CANADENSIS

Also known as	Yellow root
Where found	Cultivated in North America
Appearance	Tall-growing herb with disagreeable odour
Part used	Rhizome

Therapeutic uses	An excellent herb for treating gastric and skin diseases. It is particularly soothing to the epithelium – the skin surface both outside and inside the body, including mouth, throat, stomach and intestinal lining. It is antiseptic, laxative and purifies the blood. As a tonic it helps those with irritable and inflammatory conditions of the gastrointestinal tract. It is indicated in most digestive disorders.
Prepared as	Decoction, powder, tincture, lotion.

Hops
HUMULUS LUPULUS

Where found	Cultivated in most parts of the world.
Appearance	A climbing vine
Part used	Strobiles
Therapeutic uses	A nervine tonic and sedative mainly used in combination with other remedies for indigestion and as a liver and gall bladder remedy. It allays pain and promotes restful sleep.
Prepared as	Infusion, tincture.

Lady's Slipper
CYPRIPEDIUM PUBESCENS

Also known as	Nerve Root
Where found	Europe and the United States.
Appearance	A delicate wild orchid at present in short supply and, therefore, expensive. Attempts to grow it commercially for medicinal use have not been very successful.
Part used	Rhizome
Therapeutic uses	A most effective nervine used to allay disorders of a nervous origin, including emotional tension and hysteria. It helps to induce natural sleep. It is also antispasmodic and relaxing. A useful treatment for menopausal problems, anxiety states, spontaneous seminal emissions, excessive sexual desire, painful periods.
Prepared as	Powder, decoction, fluid extract, tincture.

Lemon Balm
MELISSA OFFICINALIS

Also known as	Sweet Balm.
Where found	A common garden herb.
Appearance	It belongs to the nettle family to which it bears some resemblance, but has a strong lemon smell.

Parts used	Leaves, whole herb.
Therapeutic uses	Carminative. A useful and safe remedy in flatulence and gastric disturbances. It has intestinal antifungal properties and is also indicated in fevers. It will induce sweating. An infusion of the leaves (one ounce to one pint of boiling water) can be drunk freely.
Prepared as	Infusion, tincture

Marshmallow
ALTHAEA OFFICINALIS

Also known as	Schloss tea
Where found	Throughout Europe
Appearance	A strong-growing herb usually found in watery places
Parts used	Leaves and root
Therapeutic uses	An emollient and demulcent; soothing to the gastrointestinal tract. Used in irritable and ulcerative conditions. An excellent treatment in cystitis and is an important ingredient in cough mixtures.
Prepared as	Infusion (of leaves), decoction (of root), syrup, tincture, poultice.

Poplar
POPULUS TREMULOIDES

Also known as	Quaking aspen
Where found	North America and Europe
Appearance	A large tree
Part used	Bark
Therapeutic uses	A tonic that improves appetite and digestion and helps to dispel flatulence. A useful medicine to take during convalescence following a fever. It is indicated in diarrhoea. Poplar has also been found to be beneficial in cases of muscular rheumatism and arthritis.
Prepared as	Decoction, powder, tincture

Prickly Ash
XANTHOXYLUM AMERICANUM

Also known as	Toothache tree
Where found	Canada and the United States
Appearance	Medium-sized tree
Parts used	Bark and berries
Therapeutic uses	The berries are carminative – they help ease griping pains in the gastrointestinal tract, expel flatulence and reduce distension. Also helpful as a circulatory tonic and treatment for chronic rheumatism.
Prepared as	Decoction, fluid extract and tincture.

Pulsatilla
ANEMONE PULSATILLA

Also known as	Wild flower
Where found	Britain and Europe
Part used	Leaves
Therapeutic uses	Sedative, nervine, antispasmodic. Helpful for women with menstrual problems and also for headaches associated with tension. Also indicated for insomnia and skin eruptions
Prepared as	Infusion, tincture.

Raspberry
RUBUS IDAEUS

Where found	Common in gardens in most temperate climates.
Appearance	A bush producing edible fruit
Part used	Leaves
Therapeutic uses	Astringent and stimulant. A useful remedy for simple diarrhoea in children. It is mild in action and soothing to the mucous lining of the intestinal tract. A gargle is used to soothe sore throats. The hormone-like action of raspberry tea explains its traditional use for easier and speedier labour in childbirth and as a remedy for painful periods.

| **Prepared as** | Infusion (which may be used as a gargle, lotion, and douche), tincture. |

Red Sage
SALVIA OFFICINALIS

Also known as	Garden sage
Where found	Commonly cultivated as a culinary herb in Europe and the United States
Appearance	A herb growing to about 12cm with purplish flowers
Part used	Leaves
Therapeutic uses	An astringent with stimulating and carminative properties. Useful in dyspepsia and flatulence and for those with poor digestion in debilitated conditions. The infusion is also used as a gargle in sore throat, quinsy and laryngitis. It also helps prevent excessive perspiration.
Prepared as	Infusion, tincture.

Rosemary
ROSMARINUS OFFICINALIS

| **Where found** | A well known garden herb |
| **Appearance** | A shrubby herb with evergreen spiky leaves and small pale blue flowers |

Part used	Leaves
Therapeutic uses	Stomachic and nervine. Indicated in headaches due to gastric disturbance. It is also carminative and antifungal. A few leaves infused in a cup of boiling water for two minutes is the best way to take it. It is also used externally in hair lotions and shampoos, probably because in the past it had a reputation for preventing baldness
Prepared as	Infusion, oil

Senna
CASSIA ANGUSTIFOLIA

Where found	Egypt, Sudan, India
Appearance.	A shrub with greyish-green winged leaves
Parts used	Leaves, pods
Therapeutic uses	Laxative and cathartic. It is given when it is necessary to clear the large intestine rapidly of faecal matter. Combine with aromatic herbs such as Cloves, Ginger, Cinnamon or Aniseed to prevent griping pains.
Prepared as	Decoction, infusion, syrup, fluid extract, tincture. Not recommended in inflammatory bowel conditions.

Stone Root
COLLINSONIA CANADENSIS

Also known as	Heal-all
Where found	Canada
Appearance	Woodland plant with large greenish-yellow flowers
Part used	Root
Therapeutic uses	Gastrointestinal tonic and antispasmodic indicated in gastroenteritis and haemorrhoids. It is also diuretic and helpful in most urinary tract complaints
Prepared as	Decoction, tincture.

Thyme
THYMUS VULGARIS

Where found	Common garden plant
Appearance	Small perennial herb with tiny leaves
Part used	Herb
Therapeutic uses	Antispasmodic and tonic. Contains thymol, a strong antiseptic, useful in irritable coughs and catarrh
Prepared as	Infusion is sweetened with honey and given in tablespoonful doses.

Valerian
VALERIAN OFFICINALIS

Also known as	All heal

Where found	Near streams, rivers and ditches in Britain
Appearance	Grows to about a metre in height with pinkish white flowers
Part used	Rhizome
Therapeutic uses	Nervine, sedative and antispasmodic. Combined with ginger for the treatment of abdominal colic and cramps, stomach pains and diarrhoea. Excellent for relieving nervous tension and debility. Promotes sleep.
Prepared as	Decoction, fluid extract, tincture.

Vervain
VERBENA OFFICINALIS

Also known as	Herb of Grace
Where found	By roadside and in meadows in Britain
Appearance	A perennial trailing herb bearing small pale-lilac flowers
Part used	Leaves
Therapeutic uses	Antispasmodic, blood purifier and tonic. It improves liver function and clears mucous from the digestive canal. It is also an excellent nervine helping to lift depression and ease tension
Prepared as	Infusion, tincture.

81

Wild Yam
DIOSCOREA VILLOSA

Also known as	Colic Root
Where found	Tropical countries, United States and Canada
Appearance	A perennial climbing plant
Part used	Root
Therapeutic uses	An antispasmodic and relaxant useful for neuralgia, bilious colic, flatulence, nausea of pregnancy, spasmodic asthma, cramping pains, painful periods, uterine pain, and rheumatism arising from liver and digestive disorders
Prepared as	Decoction, fluid extract, tincture. Note: dried root quickly loses its therapeutic potency.

Witch Hazel
HAMAMELIS VIRGINIANA

Where found	United States and Canada
Appearance	Similar to an apple tree
Parts used	Bark and leaves
Therapeutic uses	An astringent, tonic and sedative. A valuable remedy in diarrhoea and dysentery, mucous discharge and bleeding from the intestinal canal. A remedy for painful, bleeding piles
Prepared as	Decoction, tincture, distilled water, ointment, suppositories.

Wood Betony
BETONICA OFFICINALIS

Also known as   Bishopswort

Where found   Woodland in Europe

Appearance   A broad-leaved plant with spikes of red flowers spotted white

Parts used   Leaves, or whole herb

Therapeutic uses A general tonic particularly useful for conditions involving both nerves and stomach, such as gastralgia and headaches due to gastrointestinal disorders. Helps alleviate dyspepsia

Prepared as   Decoction, infusion, tincture

Yarrow
ACHILLEA MILLEFOLIUM

Also known as   Nosebleed, Milfoil, Thousand-leaf

Where found   Roadsides, meadows and waste ground in Britain

Appearance   An upright plant growing to about 61cm with leaves divided into a multitude of parts, hence the name thousand-leaf. The flowers are white or pink with yellowish centres.

Part used   Herb

Therapeutic uses   Astringent and diaphoretic. In gastrointestinal disease it is indicated in chronic diarrhoea with bleeding. Also used for bleeding piles. It stimulates the appetite and tones the digestive tract. Its diaphoretic property makes it an excellent remedy in colds, flu and catarrh: combine with peppermint.

Prepared as   Cold infusion, hot infusion (for colds), tincture.

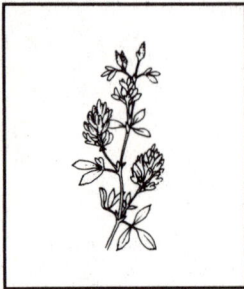

Lucerne

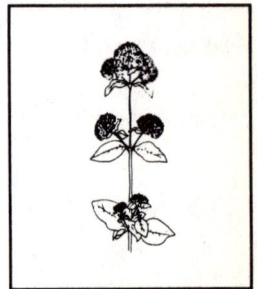

Marjoram, Sweet

Chapter 15

Vitamin and Mineral Therapy

Vitamin and mineral supplementation can be a useful adjunctive therapy in some patients.

Vitamin C aids normal bowel function and, when taken in megadoses (1g daily), can effectively relieve constipation.

Diarrhoea, constipation and other bowel symptoms, including flatulence, distension, badly-smelling stools and weak abdominal muscles can be due to a deficiency of dietary magnesium. Taking a magnesium supplement or magnesium-rich foods will, therefore, help constipation in these cases. Among fruits rich in magnesium are: apples, grapes, pears, oranges, grapefruit, lemons, cherries, peaches and plums.

JUICES

A fruit and vegetable juicer is a useful health appliance. Freshly extracted juices are full of minerals and vitamins and not only are a great boost to recovery from disease, but taken on a daily basis will help to maintain health. A wineglassful before each meal is about the right amount to take.

For constipation use carrot juice and apple, separately or combined, or tomato, celery and radish. For diarrhoea use carrot, apple and celery, or carrot and celery with a smaller amount of spinach and parsley juice added. Spinach and parsley juices are very potent and are best not taken on their own. For a bowel tonic use a cocktail of orange juice, carrot and spinach.

Chapter 16

Seeking Professional Help

Although this book is aimed at giving those with irritable bowel syndrome information and guidance on treatment with herbal medicines and diet, it cannot be stressed too much that quicker results can often be achieved by consulting a fully qualified herbal or naturopathic practitioner.

Patients are seen by appointment and in confidence in the practitioner's consulting rooms. Herbal practitioners qualified with the National Institute of Medical Herbalists, can be recognised by the initials MNIMH or FNIMH after their names. They are trained to deal with a wide range of medical problems, although some practitioners may specialise in certain medical areas.

Naturopaths trained at the British College of Naturopathy and Osteopathy in London and admitted to the Register of Naturopaths have the letters ND MRN after their names. They are specialists in the non-drug treatment of a wide variety of conditions, although many naturopaths specialise in musculoskeletal problems.

The National Institute of Medical Herbalists, founded in 1864, is the oldest established body of practising medical herbalists in the world. Members can be found in most towns in the UK. The easiest way to find out if there is one near you is to look under 'Herbalists' in Yellow Pages, Thomson's, or other local directory.

The aim of both naturopathy and herbal medicine is not just to relieve symptoms but to offer the sufferer an increased level of general health. The practitioner takes an holistic approach to his patients, an approach that is being followed more and more by other primary health care practitioners.

He will, therefore, take into account not only the physical symptoms of irritable bowel syndrome but also any mental stress or emotional problems which may be relevant.

Both the body and the mind conform to the laws of nature, one of the most important of which is the law of homoeostasis – the ability of the individual to be self-regulating, despite changes in the environment.

It is the law of balance that has enabled us to survive for thousands of years despite changes, or threats, in the environment, whether it be a simple change in temperature, or an infection due to pathogenic micro-organisms.

Disease is produced when outside threats, or changes, are too overwhelming and the individual fails to respond or adapt healthily.

Many bowel problems can be traced back to imbalances in the individual's early family life.

It is not always easy to treat oneself appropriately. It quite often needs a trained practitioner to give guidance so that the deeper reasons for an illness and not just the superficial are treated.

YOUR STORY

Readers who have benefited from the use of herbal medicine, for any condition, either from home use or from those prescribed by professional medical herbalists, are invited to send details to the author of this series of books, c/o the publishers, W. Foulsham & Co. Ltd, Yeovil Road, Slough, Berkshire SL1 4JH. Unfortunately, the author regrets that he is unable to enter into any correspondence on this matter.

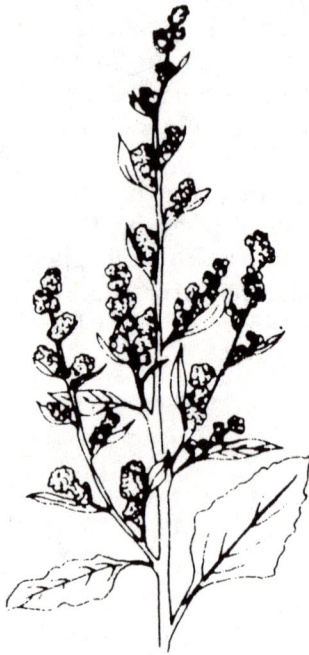

Glossary of common medical terms

Very often when reading, or on having a medical consultation, words are used which may not be familiar. This short list will help to make some of the more common ones a little clearer.

Alterative
A medicine that beneficially alters the condition of a patient. In herbal medicine it usually refers to a remedy that purifies the blood by improving the function of the organs, such as liver and kidneys, which are involved in this process.

Amenorrhoea
Absence of menstrual periods.

Anodyne
A medicine that alleviates pain – physical or mental.

Analgesic
A medicine that blocks pain.

Anthelmintic
A medicine that is used to rid the body of intestinal worms.

Antiseptic
A medicine, or other substance, that prevents putrefaction.

Antispasmodic
A remedy that prevents or relieves spasms.

Aperient
A remedy that produces a natural movement of the bowels.

Aphrodisiac
A substance that produces sexual desire and stimulates the sexual organs.

Astringent
Binding or contracting tissues.

Cardiac	Relating to the heart, either a medicine, or disease, that alters heart function.
Carminative	A medicine that eases griping pains and flatulence in the bowel.
Cathartic	A strong laxative, or purgative, producing evacuation of the bowel.
Corrective	Correcting or counteracting the harmful and restoring to a healthy state.
Debility	Feebleness of health; run down.
Degenerative	A disease that results in destruction or disintegration of tissue.
Demulcent	A soothing medicine, mostly applied to those that act on the gastrointestinal canal.
Deobstruent	Removing obstructions and opening the ducts and other natural passages of the body.
Diaphoretic	A substance that induces perspiration.
Diuretic	A substance that increases the flow of urine.
Dysmenorrhoea	Excessive pain during menstruation.
Emetic	Any substance that causes vomiting.
Emmenagogue	A remedy that brings on the menstrual period.
Emollient	A medicine that softens, soothes and lubricates skin and internal tissues.
Haemostatic	A substance that checks bleeding and aids clotting of the blood.

Insecticide	Any substance that is fatal to insects.
Laxative	A substance that induces gentle, and easy bowel movement.
Leucorrhoea	A mucous discharge from the female genital organs, previously known as "the whites".
Menorrhagia	Excessive flow of menstrual blood.
Myalgia	Muscular pain; muscular rheumatism.
Narcotic	A drug that produces drowsiness, sleep, stupor and insensibility.
Nephritic	Relating to the kidneys.
Nervine	A remedy that relieves a nerve disorder and restores the nervous system to its normal state.
Oxytocic	A drug that causes contractions of the uterus and hastens childbirth.
Parturient	A remedy used during childbirth.
Purgative	A medicine taken to evacuate the bowels, but one that is much stronger that a laxative or aperient.
Resolvent	A drug, application, or other substance that reduces swellings and tumours.
Rubefacient	A treatment that produces redness, inflammation and blisters of the skin; a counter-irritant (rubefy = make red).
Sedative	A remedy soothing to the nervous system; a tranquilliser.
Soporific	Promoting sleep.

Stimulant   A remedy that produces a rapid increase in vital energy of part or of the whole body.

Stomachic   Relating to the stomach; a remedy that aids the normal function of the stomach, promoting proper digestion and appetite.

Styptic   A substance that checks bleeding.

Sudorific   A remedy that produces heavy perspiration.

Tonic   A medicine that invigorates or tones up a part or the whole of the body and promotes wellbeing.

Vermifuge   A medicine that expels worms from the body.

Vulnerary   An ointment or treatment that promotes the healing of wounds.

FURTHER READING

Other books in this herbal series include:

Skin Problems
Arthritis and Rheumatism
Stress and Nervous Tension
Sexual Problems.

The Author

David Potterton is a consultant medical herbalist and registered naturopath with practices in Reading and Wokingham, Berkshire.

He is a member of the National Institute of Medical Herbalists (NIMH) and of the British Naturopathic Association (BNA). He is also a member of the General Council and Register of Naturopaths.

Mr Potterton has been a member of the McCarrison Society –a medical organisation devoted to the study of health and nutrition – for many years.

He was previously a member of the Royal Society of Medicine and a member of the Vegetarian Society's research committee.

Mr Potterton has been tutor in materia medica and in pathology for the NIMH, and has conducted a series of further education lecture courses on herbal medicine for Berkshire County Council. He also lectures frequently to local organisations in the Thames Valley.

As a writer, Mr Potterton has contributed to all the major health magazines in the UK, including "Here's Health" and "Healthy Living", and was the English editor of "Bestways", the American health magazine, as well as being a contributor to the "US Quarterly Journal of Health".

He was medical editor of the family doctor newspaper "Doctor" for many years, and co-editor of the "British Journal of Phytotherapy", a professional journal for herbal practitioners and naturopathic physicians both in the UK and abroad.

He is the editor of several books published by Foulsham, including "Culpeper's Colour Herbal" and "Medicinal Plants". He has revised and edited a series of books by herbalist Mervyn Mitton on: "Arthritis and Rheumatism", "Skin Problems" and "Stress and Tension".